MW01233843

Potty Training Strategies

Everything a Parent Needs to Know to Get His Toddler Diaper Free Quickly and Without Stress in 3 Easy Steps

Written By

Jennifer Siegel

Table of Contents

INTRODUCTION

Thank you for purchasing this book!

Parental Guidance For Potty Training

Parents can prepare their kids before they're ready. After my surprise with my first toddler telling me it's time, and I started preparing the next one. Talking to your toddler about how regular these movements are and allowing them to watch you on the big toilet can start this process. Ask them a question every time you change their diaper. Honey, you made a big pee pee today. You can tell Mommy when you're ready to throw these diapers away. We can buy you a fancy new potty when you're ready." Keep reminding them so that they tell you when the time comes. They might even use body cues when they gently pinch their legs to show you when the time has come.

Play games with them to teach them some physical cues. Help them to point to body parts and name them. Show your two-year-old some cute undies they can wear and show them that you wear these undies too. Let them feel how light and soft it is compared to a wet, soggy diaper. Don't expect anything from them, but introduce them to the freedom of undies slowly for short periods. This also starts building communication between you for potty training. Tell your little one that you must pee-pee and head off to the toilet. Allow them to be curious and follow you. The rule here is that dads teach boys and moms teach girls to avoid confusion about body parts.

A "game on" secret: Another show and tell exercise is to play potty with a doll or their favorite teddy bear. Take your toddler into the bathroom and talk them through how the doll uses the potty. "Teddy is going to the potty now. He pulls down his undies and sits comfortably. He can read a book while he waits to pee. He can also sing a song. Wow, Teddy had made a pee-pee in the potty. Teddy wipes himself with toilet paper. Now he must flush the old food down the toilet." Be descriptive and turn this into a fun show and tell. The trick here is to start asking your toddler to fill in the gaps. "What must Teddy do next?" You know that Teddy must wash his hands, but you want your toddler to say it after a few shows.

Enjoy your reading!

Potty Training Seats-Pros And Cons Investigation

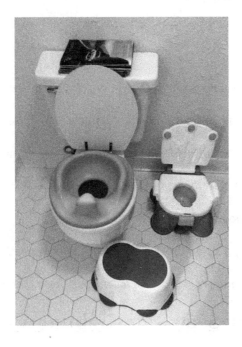

Today, many parents opt only for a potty toilet when their child is trained.

A potty seat is a small seat that fits on an adult toilet and thereby eliminates the need to empty the bowl of a potted chair.

Instead of using a potty chair in the bathroom, there are both advantages and drawbacks to training your child, and we shall discuss the difference in its post.

Potty Seats For Training-Pros

Chapter 1: The most apparent benefit of using a toilet is the one already mentioned. When your baby sits on the top of an adult pot, all waste enters the adult toilet directly. Do not spill, tip over, cleans, smell et al., with a potty chair bowl.

Chapter 2: By using a potty seat, you're never going to have to change the position from a potty chair. He has the adult toilet from the get-go entirely comfortably.

Chapter 3: There is a portable toilet training seat. Only throw one into your car, and you always have the right potty in size anywhere an adult toilet is located for your preschooler or infant.

Chapter 4: A potty seat also makes a baby feel big automatically, as she knows that the adults use only the adult's toilet. She's doing that now.

Potty Seats For Training-Cons

Chapter 5: The problem of safety can be linked to potty seats. For the child to climb on the training sit safely, you must have some step stool. Some kids like it, but some kids don't like Its area very much because they are quite afraid of using a toilet. A frightened kid doesn't practice well potty if or not.

Chapter 6: In the way can be potty chairs each time an adult needs to use the bathroom, and you must push it. Of course, if your child is new to training, you may want to remove the adult toilet seat because accidents can and do occur when a child attempts to lay the potted seat on an adult toilet or wait for assistance.

Chapter 7: A potty seat needs to provide a room for your child to firmly place his foot so that it can pass through the intestine. The floor immediately does it on a potty chair. Often, the step height is the same for a potty seat, but often, when a child is seated, the step height is not right.

Chapter 8: An adult toilet training chair is not suitable for young boys who want to be standing and choosing like papa. Think of how you want to train your son toilet before reaching a potty seat automatically.

Potty training seats are an excellent convenience for potty boys if appropriately used. Many parents follow a world-famous trend, use a potty chair, and then move to a potty seat when they get older.

In the end? Choosing a potty toilet seat depends on your toilet training method and your child's unique personality. Individual parents are glad to have both a potty seat and a potty chair, and some potty chairs are separated to be used as both a chair and stool. A parent must also be flexible because a child can favor one or another child and then change his or her mind as he or she progresses into age and maturity.

It makes your child's experience so potable as possible is the most crucial factor to consider. You want to know that the potty chair or seat that you choose does its job by being safe, comfortable, and in keeping with your home life. The training process is based on the integration of ups and downs and what you most want is to know.

Potty Chairs-How To Select The Right Person

You certainly have seen potty training chairs as you are planning to educate your child shortly.

Don't You Have Many Choices?

Elegant, simple, one-piece, hand-paint, multipurpose, gender, and portable for beginners.

Since you have possibly declined to buy one of these items, how do you determine which one or two work best for your child?

It is a great question. It is a great question. Consider several kinds of potty chairs and see the main advantages of using them.

Small Potty Or Potty Seat Training Chair.

First of all, you have to determine whether you want to have a potty chair (a toilet with a children's bathroom on the ground) or a potty (a children's bathroom seat on an adult bathroom).

A potty seat may not have to replace the potty bowl (sounding good), but you need to remember that many kids don't mount the grownup toilet comfortably from the room.

Specific To Gender-Or Not.

Some potty chairs are suitable for boys or girls, but some are specially made for only one sex.

Frankly, as those pots work all right, you run the risk of getting another potty the next time you intend on having more than one boy. Splash guards are things to watch for that are high enough for small boys, but it is easy to stride for both boys and girls. Many spritz guards may be disabled for young girls, but watch the guard off for sharp edges.

A Bowl Or A Single Plate.

One-piece, accessible to vacuum, is the best potty chair. They are smart and circular – no borders to pinch small thighs.

However, other parents, like myself, want a potty bowl to be removed. That means the potty chair has something else to scrub, but it is well worth it if you empty the potty for months a couple of times a day.

Seek a bowl that can also be quickly removed. All the better if you can do it all on your own. You would finally want your baby to do the job by himself, but you don't like something complicated or easy to spill over.

15

Handheld Pots And Fly.

After potty training with my own four girls, I can tell you if you want to suggest going to your car for a journey or a portable potty-training chair.

Instead, irrespective of how hot a public toilet is (or whether it is not at all available), potty training is continuing. You can get cuddly chairs, have liners on them, or even use the whole potty chair.

You can also get folding potty seats on public adult toilets to help your young child feel safe and comfortable.

Potties Specialization.

These are the potty stalls that are fun. You can have musical potties (such as playing music when a sensor senses wetness, others can force your kid to play a song), potty characters, and hand-painted potty chairs that are lovely rocker chairs when you have potty training.

I Was Summing Up.

Bear in mind how you want to train and the personality of your child when shopping for potty training chairs. You clean a lot, and your kid must feel comfortable and motivated while using it.

Between these potty chairs, there are no wrong or correct choices. In each of your home bathrooms, you may need one, and in the car, you need one.

Or you can decide that the best option for your family is a simple potty seat that can be branded anywhere you go.

Everything's good. The crucial thing is to keep potty exercises up-to-date while you and your child move together on its significant milestone.

Potty Training Aids.

You've already looked at the dizzying variety of potty-training aids available today on the market, whether you're already in potty education with a baby or preschool.

Or have you ever seen how many different styles of cupid chairs exist, be it potatoes, stickers, books, photos, goals, watches, seats, or chairs?

The real question is, the toiletries do you need to train your child?

Here Is An Explanation Of Some Of The Various Potty Aids Currently Available And For Which They Are Helpful.

Limited Sunsets.

Start the big one. Let's start the big one. Potty chairs. Potty chairs. You're going to want to clean something safe and secure. If you train a kid, a splash guard is right. Beyond that, it depends on you and your child's personal preferences.

You can take your child to shop for his new potty chair with you if you like, or you can think about his temperament and choose what you know is going to work with him. Character sessions, musical sessions, potty chairs, and multipurpose chairs are available.

The portable or travel potty is one kind of chair you want to remember. Confide in me, and there are occasions when it is crucial, as the park without toilets, the filthy public bathroom, or just driving down the road when your kid can no longer wait.

Potty seats, as potty chairs, are unique. They are children's seats, which fit on top of the toilets of adult height. Some kids climb a stepping stool to go on top and do their business while being convenient to use. Personally, after their toilet training, my kids used It special potty-training aid.

Potty Dolls. -Potty Dolls.

The IF can be useful for training dolls correctly. A real potty exercise doll takes water and then "pees" on-demand, showing your kid exactly how you expect it. Its clarity is often sufficient to train some kids.

You may opt to use a favorite doll or stuffed home animal and pretend to use potty items. It helps a great many children, especially those who understand the potty process already. Consider your child and his style of learning to see whether a potty doll is useful in your home.

Books And Videos.

A selection of these probably come from you. Start to learn what is available in your local library. First of all, read and watch without your child to make sure the message conveyed suits your child's needs.

Books and videos are potty training aids frequently used by infants, which make them strong by repetition. So, pick those that you can still read/see! Nice if you have a dumb potty or dance; these are perfect instruments to hold your young potty trainee.

Watches And Targets.

Potty goals are flushable things in the toilet and let your child shoot and aim. As you can imagine, at least at first, these are so much fun and inspiring. They seem to lose their luster quickly, so I suggest that they are held for individual therapies or if a child needs support for an extended period.

Tight watches are a device you can use to help your preschooler take care of themselves. For 60 or 90 minutes, you decide if you want your child to use the bowl, and you set the time on the watch. When it's time for the potty, the clock vibrates or plays music. It can help you stop stuttering and encourage your child to pay more attention.

Stamps, Cookies, Trophies.

It is using such potty helpers and a potty reward map to help your child envision its success in potty training. Generally speaking, it is a good idea to change charts and prizes to avoid frustration. (by the way, keep the rewards small).

In short, it is one of the best and useful tools available for potty training. Think of your child's personality and personal preferences, and you be able to make the right decision to begin the potty-training process with your child.

Nighttime Training

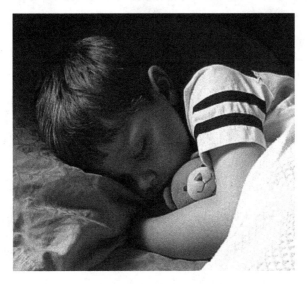

Nighttime training is more challenging because it depends on your child's ability to hold the urine for an extended duration and how deeply s/he sleeps. The urge to go might be severe for them to notice when sleeping, so getting up in the middle of the night might not take place.

Start by restricting fluid intake right before bed. While some people do not feel like It ought to be done, the reality is that if there's absolutely nothing in their little body to expel, they not go. If you haven't ended night bottles, now is most likely the time to do so.

Don't deny a thirsty kid a beverage of water. Some states that were going to bed hungry repair a child's mind on the water and increase the possibilities of nighttime wetting.

Keep bedtime calm. The threat of bedwetting can be increased if your kid takes part in great deals of roughhousing or even an exciting TV program near to bedtime. When kids are delighted, they tend to produce more urine. Keep her/him calm by having a peaceful discussion or checking out a story to her/him.

Before your kid goes to sleep, have her shot to go to the bathroom one more time. Even if she states, she does not attempt anyhow. Your child might say something; however, when they rest on the potty, they go!

Think about not using training trousers at night. Although you did not plan it, continuing to put your child in training trousers for bedtime and expecting her not to have "accidents" might be sending her a mixed message. Initially, you need to most likely begin with a diaper in the evening with praise in the early morning for a dry diaper. However, right after that, please put them in regular underwear at bedtime.

Be alert for unforeseen nightly sees. While your child gets used to underwear in the evening, s/he may have a mishap, and after that, get up before you do. She or he be unpleasant and either call out to you or get out of bed and pay you a checkout.

Make sure the way to the bathroom is lit, even if only with night-lights. Draw a map with your child showing how from the bed to the restroom to help form a visual image. You may wish to purchase an automated sensor light in the bathroom that comes on automatically when somebody enters the room.

Keep your home warm enough so the kid won't avoid getting up because it's too cold. You can return to energy savings later on.

Think about keeping a potty chair near your kid's bed if that makes things easier.

Practice "favorable picturing" as you put your kid to sleep. Assist a kid picture remaining dry all night and getting up dry in the morning. Talk about the enjoyment of feeling dehydrated, in control, and developed.

Try whispering "dry" concepts into the ear of a sleeping kid. It is something psychologists say children are typically receptive to such "concept planting" throughout specific periods of sleep.

Let your child know that you understand that he or she remains dry during the night soon," like other big kids. It is essential to establish the expectation, but do not subject your child to heavy pressure.

Please remove diapers and change them with training pants, fabric soakers, or nonreusable pull-ups only after a week or so of dry nights.

If your kid does have a mishap, try not to make a big deal about it. Reassure them that accidents do occur. Some psychologists advise having the kid clean up their mess. It consists of stripping the bed and positioning the stained sheets in the laundry bin and putting brand-new sheets on the bed.

Its whole procedure, do not concentrate on the mishap and do not make your kid feel guilty for having an accident.

A plastic sheet under the regular sheets also assists you to save the mattress.

Nighttime dryness does not always instantly follow day time dryness and could typically use up to a couple of months or even years. Practice persistence and make sure that there isn't a healing factor for its issue.

Another problem throughout toilet training is how to preserve development while traveling.

Potty Training Aids: Modern And Traditional

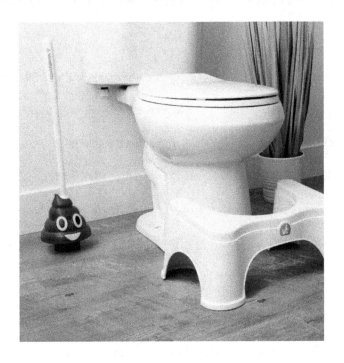

There are many aids to potty training today as we are a globalized community with zillions of options for each reaction, stimuli, and action regarding newborn and baby-care. Potty training techniques and methods are as diverse as the populous on earth itself. Let us hence start with the very history of potty training.

History Of Potty Training

The approach towards potty training was completely parent-centric as the cleaning up after and during the use of diapers would be reduced if the child were trained to potty.

Usually, mothers would force kids to sit on a comfortable and makeshift potty seat periodically that the child is acquainted with as potty time. While cloth diapers were always accessible, with the growing age of a child, it was thought that potty training is healthy. Some parents let their children relieve themselves in public, while some do not. It is always good to provide a hygienic and fearless space for your child to facilitate himself or herself while in the act of it.

Generally, parents picked up a child's cues to interest in the bathroom and other signs to potty comfortable, private, and safe. History says that parents have been harsh in teaching anything to kids, but potty training should be conducted fearlessly and in love. History shows many parents taking their kids to relive out in nature, before the advent of cabins called bathrooms. Cleaning the private parts in the water alongside the baby's father or mother undoubtedly be ideal for teaching potty training. Be alert to ensure that your baby is hygienic around the potty as some kids tend to mess with the excreta. Hence, be harsh about how dangerous, toxic, and dirty excreta are to your baby!

Traditional Aids To Train, Your Baby To Healthy Potty

1. Potty out in nature: traditionally, as aforementioned, relieving yourself in nature helped a parent communicate through practical means in training a child to potty.

2. Potty together: when a child is taught to pee or poop alongside a parent who demonstrates and helps the child to it, the child gets the real way of following the act.

3. Disciplined potty training: with families more than 2-3 kids, there were harsh means of old potty training, where an ordinary potty training person usually trained kids. The punishments were severe, and the rules strict. Kids are put through regular practice and discipline to communicate and follow potty training methods in their case.

4. Clothes or diapers: clothes were bundled up, to pose as diapers in older times, for a baby. However, washing and hygiene of these cloths were always skeptical. As materials were not disposable, a baby could develop many rashes through the unchanged diaper.

5. Naked Hours: another easy way to teach your baby to potty is through the act of open hours. When a child feels peeing or pooping while naked, his or her little palm was not enough to stop the flow of Nature. It

incapability of stopping to pee or poo teach the baby to run to the bathroom beforehand. If the baby is naked, parents can, at all times, observe the cleanliness and comfort of their little one.

6. Potty bell: another essential and useful potty training technique is the help of a potty training bell. Potty bells are used to make a routine drill or practice for potty training. It can also habituate a kid to go to the bathroom eventually when the bell rings.

7. Rewards: always make sure that you reward your baby for his or her well and disciplined behavior. Only when you acknowledge and emphasize the baby know that he or she has done something good or something that should be repeated.

Modern Ways To Potty Training

Today, there are many aids available to help a parent train their little one to the potty system. Some are:

1. Potty Seats: these are comfortable and snug seats to keep your baby's vulnerable and tender body from touching the dirty toilets. Parents can also use a portable toilet to empty the contents into the bathroom later on. Potty seats should be chosen after you check with the measurements of your baby. It should never be too loose or tight for the babe.

2. Potty training dolls: another great toy that is beneficial to a baby is the potty training dolls. A parent can use a child's favorite toy and demonstrate ways to potty with it.

3. Potty training videos: Many child specialists have provided descriptive and useful videos for potty training your little one. Research, check, and buy these modern aids for potty training!

4. Potty training professionals: today, you even have experienced people or professionals who can help you train your kid to potty in healthy and hygienic ways.

5. Disposable diapers: another essential aspect of natural substitute for potty training is the disposable and safe diapers with sturdy hold. Use it until your child can walk, after which, potty training is a comfortable bathroom should be trained.

6. Musical influence: another remarkable discovery of the age is soothing music for the baby while peeing or pooping. It reduces fear in your baby during the same.

7. Games for potty practice: practice duration of pooping, peeing and aiming into the closet, and number of poops and other healthy and hygienic games to promote your baby to poop whenever he or she feels like.

8. Potty training celebration: conduct potty training drills and events to improve proper potty training with the family's help.

Potty Training: Merits And Harms

Diapers Or Direct To The Bathroom?

The question has its answer for both a settled parent and a hurrying parent. Potty training has its long-term and deep-rooted benefits to both the child and the parents. On the other hand, the wrong side of potty training can also result in long-term damage to the baby's mental and physical setup. Hence, potty training requires thorough care, alertness, and education to be started. Primarily, one should be aware of the merits of potty training for both parents and the baby.

Merits Of Potty Training

1. Promote activity in your baby: your baby becomes aware of potty training times and drills, so he or she runs to the toilet, hearing the potty bell or with you, while you're off to pee! To promote potty training as a fun activity, make your baby practice pooping or peeing as mock drills as well. It boosts his or her healthy metabolism and overcoming the diaper aspects of laziness. Movement and growth as inter-related for a newborn, and parents should be well aware of spending productive and progressive time with their babies.

2. Promote hygiene: one of the most important aspects of potty training is that it promotes the reason and comfort of keeping a healthy, clean, and

hygienic care about one's private and public space. The earlier it is instilled in a child, the better! A child learns to keep him or her clean, fragrant, and hygienic at all times of his waking and resting hours.

3. Promote a healthy diet: with potty training comes keeping or watching the food of your baby and starting him or her on the route to the ritual of brushing and freshening up in the morning together with parents!

4. Promotes self-control: healthy potty-trained child always has high self-control skills; with lessons of being aware of peeing and pooping a minute before the water or the solid hits the bottom, your baby acquires skills of controlling or exercising his or her voluntary power on the body. It adds a bit of consciousness education on your baby's psyche as well.

5. Promotes alertness and awareness: with the growing knowledge of his or her time and space, the baby becomes alert and aware of his or her surroundings; potty training makes a child become alert himself or herself about others' habits and mannerisms as well.

6. Promotes social skills: proper potty training also instills habits of active social skills in your baby; your baby starts to behave, imitate, and communicate with his or her society in a style or way that he or she is comfortable with.

7. Promotes independence and confidence: a baby who is trained healthy in the forefront of the potty is also independent; he or she is confident about his behavior, hygiene, fragrance, and air, in the able actuality.

8. Economically profitable: another important thing is to, indeed, save on those diapers!

Disadvantages Of Improper Potty Training

The demerits of improper or unhygienic potty training result in an adverse outcome harmful to your baby's physical and mental setup. Some of these are long-term and short-term. They are:

1. Rashes: firstly, if the private parts are not taken care of well, the baby develops rashes and allergies in his or her private areas. These can result from inadequate water, dryness, and other chemical reactions on your baby's skin.

2. Infections: rashes and other prolonged negligence for hygienic potty training result in severe diseases and degenerations.

3. Gastrointestinal disorders: babies tend to develop many digestive disorders in the first few years of their vulnerable times of immunity. Parents should observe and medicate the child sensibly to avoid painful ordeals of gastro-intestinal-disorders.

4. Fear: another vital aspect of improper or harsh potty training is that these heap up to a significant concern towards the bathroom, private areas, and excretion. It can grow into nightmares and other anti-social behavior in babies.

5. Bedwetting: another essential result of the fear above is the bedwetting by babies. Take care to wake your baby up for a bathroom break in the middle of the night. It is healthy if your baby has been wetting his or her bed frequently.

6. Lousy communication: another cause and result of improper potty training is the gap between the baby and everyone else. The baby has to be connected in the most intimate ways. It happens via healthy communication exhibited by babies resulting from faith and trust in their parents' safety and omnipotence!

7. Insomnia: a baby can end up losing sleep owing to the fear of bedwetting or such incidents.

8. Unhygienic private care: Improper potty training aids grow babies into children and them into youth with complete negligence on their hygiene and care.

Always take care to consider and seek professional help whenever you believe that you are making a breakthrough or giant leap in your baby's life. Take care.

The Power Of Feedback, The Right Way To Use Positive Reinforcement

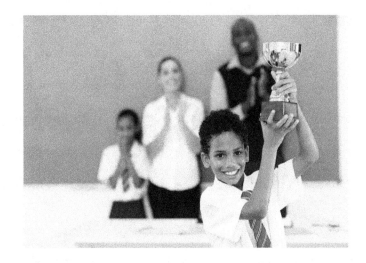

Positive Reinforcements

Q. What constitutes a positive reinforcement?

A. A positive reaction that increases the repetitiveness of the desired behavior.

Every parent knows about the importance of giving ample positive reinforcements to children. Most parents use them, whether intuitively in a completely spontaneous manner or deliberately in a calculated, deliberate way.

The intent is to use positive reinforcements as learning triggers that help children internalize desired behaviors until they own them.

What is positive reinforcement anyway? We can say that it is every pleasant consequence experienced by an individual as a direct result of It individual's behavior. In other words, when somebody does something or behaves in a certain way, positive reinforcement is an excellent outcome. Being pleasant and rewarding raises the chances that Its behavior repeats itself. Many of our actions are obtained its way the act that aroused positive reinforcement repeat itself in the future to win reinforcements once again. Therefore, we have to conclude that the support must be meaningful and significant to the receiver to maintain the receiver's motivation. Otherwise, the receiver does not care to invest efforts to win it.

Children learn how to hold their urine and BMs because uncontrolled elimination brings about unpleasant results.

They quickly learn to associate the release of urine and BMs on the carpet, floor, or clothing, with negative consequences which involve a whole array of unpleasant feelings: the wet and dirty sensation, the general unpleasantness of the situation, and adverse reactions from adults. The negative result encourages them to learn how to refrain from their kind of behavior in the future to avoid it. When on top of that, they receive a warm and reassuring reaction from meaningful adults every time success is achieved (urination and defecation in the potty or toilet), we can say that efficient, positive reinforcement has been given and that it positive encouragement is used to help them embrace a new desired habit over the old undesired one. It is how positive reinforcement impacts learning and the acquisition of new behaviors and skills.

Most sensitive and attentive parents, who know their children well, learn how to provide consistent reinforcement to win their child's attention, interest, motivation, and drive change to achieve the desired behavior.

Proper Positive Reinforcements And Bad, Positive Reinforcements

Q. How far and how long?

A. As far as you can without losing your dignity, and until the new behavior becomes second nature.

Frequency

In the beginning, it is better to provide full reinforcement, meaning that every instance in which your child behaves in the desired way should win him or her positive support with all your heart. If it follows the guidelines mentioned above, positive reinforcement contributes to a quicker and deeper internalization of a newly learned behavior.

As you progress, and after you have established that your baby or toddler demonstrates a reasonably good level of control and a high success rate, you may gradually reduce the intensity and frequency of your reinforcements. Most parents do so spontaneously and intuitively. They move from full to partial reinforcement as they go along, without giving it much thought. Partial support is reinforcement provided alternately – in some, and not all, instances of success. It is, in fact, the more common form of reinforcement used in most families' daily routines (clearly, we do not keep on praising and glorifying our children's poop until they turn eighteen). It is also the more efficient reinforcement in the long run. It promises that the desired behavior be internalized, repeated, and established.

Every time your child learns a new habit or behavior, you should begin with frequent reinforcement upon every achievement, and then lessen the frequency to partial frequency. It is not necessary to provide support every single time forever, especially since with age, more and more skills are learned, providing parents with ample opportunities to reinforce and praise their children in a wide variety of situations and achievements.

Material Reinforcement Versus Psychological Reinforcement

The major drawback when giving out material prizes is that young children quickly learn to associate positive behavior with substantial compensation or reward. These young children are liable to get a false perception of reality and conclude that every normative action on their part (which may also be positive) deserves some reward; therefore, it is worth their while to behave in the desired manner to ensure the receipt of such an award. We all realize that It is far from being true.

Another drawback would be an overturning of the situation, significantly when the process is not advancing as quickly as possible. The young child may say to his or her parents: "First, you give me my prize and then 'go' in the bathroom or toilet." These parents find themselves helpless, and more often than not, do as the child asks: provide the prize and hope for the best. But usually, the worst comes outcomes. Young children do not usually feel obliged to keep their promise if it does not serve them well. It is how the situation can get out of control quickly, while the toddler cunningly gets the upper hand of the case. The idea of the prize, which initially was supposed to function as positive reinforcement, be twisted and turned into a means of extortion. Sound cannot come out of that.

Keeping your reinforcements verbal and psychological while refraining from materiality in it respect save you much trouble. The value of verbal, mental reinforcements cannot be overestimated. We know that children, by nature, wish to please their parents. They enjoy making their parents happy and crave the feeling of pride and achievement when they succeed.

One parent told me how their child was so proud of his "creation" floating in the toilet that he demanded that it be photographed and sent immediately to daddy at work!

You must realize that alongside a childish tendency towards rebelliousness and aspiration for independence, very young children are strongly motivated towards cooperation and obedience. These traits and trends are given strong reinforcement once the parent expresses feelings of content and happiness at the child's success. Your support is all about expressions of pride and content, followed by a smile, a clap, or a cuddle. Children know how to appreciate kind words and empowering gestures, and are well aware of their role and effect on their lives. They even learn how to "embrace" themselves, and it is not unusual for young children to say the same words that they heard from their parents to themselves when circumstances justify reinforcement.

One child learned so well to provide praise that one evening, after being tucked into bed, she heard her mother come out of the bathroom and commented: "Oh, Mommy, you peed in the bathroom! Good for you! Well done!"

To conclude, let me emphasize again that positive reinforcements have an enormous impact on your child's fragile self-esteem at very young ages when it is still forming and shaping itself. Young children who internalize reinforcements are more likely to establish a positive and healthy sense of self, worth, and confidence. In later stages, children learn to internalize the positive image that their parents planted and establish for them and own it themselves. It becomes a part of them, a power they can rely on when they construct their adult personality and discover their strengths. As a result, they become less dependent on external reinforcements when they grow older. Only psychological, verbal reinforcements can do that. In other words, keep your rewards verbal, and as much as possible, do not use material ones.

Remember that material reinforcement comes and goes, and when there is too much of it, it gets less effective. On the other hand, when parents give their children emotional support, they are, in fact, "charging up" their soul and self-worth and are empowering their children to develop into healthy self-assured adults.

Keeping Reinforcement Reasonable

Beth and George ask Daphna when we began potty training, we made up the "poop song." Every time our son succeeded and pooped in the toilet, we would sing, dance, and clap our hands, which made him very happy. How long are we supposed to keep up with Its ritual? If truth is said, it's getting a little bit tiresome.

Daphna answers: If you are familiar with my doctrine, then you would know that I am all for verbal reinforcements and that I recommend avoiding material reinforcements as much as possible for fear that they morph into a very primitive form of extortion that the child learns to use on his or her parents. You have described a kind of reinforcement which probably situated on the thin line in the middle. Luckily, whereas constant support is needed in initial stages, as the baby grows more skilled, the recommendation is to tone down the intensity and the frequency of reinforcements. A partial reinforcement strategy leave room for reinforcing more new skills later on and prevent burnout of all parties involved. So, you can gradually tone down your performances until you quit them altogether. Simultaneously, progress to strictly verbal reinforcements and save them for the more challenging occasions. Before you know it, going to the toilet becomes a natural thing to do for your child, and you be reinforcing other newly-learned skills. Just a friendly suggestion: if you want to survive to parent your child until adulthood, you have to mellow down your enthusiasm somewhat and find a less exhausting form of reinforcement.

Trust Your Instincts Better Than You Trust Commercially-Interested Parties

Khara asks: Daphna, my son, has begun a weaning process. By the DVD that he watches, we've promised him a pee prize. Not only that, but we already offered and gave him stickers, chocolates, little toys, and so forth. But there seems to be no effect whatsoever on his cooperation with us in the process, and he continues to pee in his pants. What can we do?

Daphna answers: Good intentions and bad advice given by interested commercial parties led you to think that a prize overload helps you get your child to cooperate. The truth is the exact opposite. There is no more fabulous prize for a child than the right word of support, and there is no compensation higher than a hug from a content parent. Moreover, giving out the prize regardless of your child's achievements not motivate him.

Methods Of Potty Training Your Child

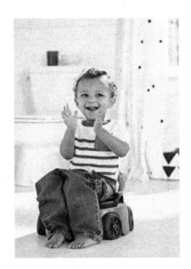

Pavlovian Potty – The Positive Reinforcement Method

As emotional beings with a need for validation, most humans – whether adults or toddlers – have been observed to perform better at tasks when rewarded with positive reinforcement. Have you noticed your child repeat a word with more enthusiasm when you clap the first time he/she said "Mama"? Has the toddler tried walking across a room more often, when encouraged by your claps and cheers? That's positive reinforcement for you – building motivation by offering encouraging rewards.

If your child responds well to a pat on the back or even a candy for a job well done, then positive reinforcement may be the simplest way to potty-train him/her. Anticipating a reward at the end of a task is often all it takes to prepare your children for days. Your child may initially use the potty to hear your cheer, but these bowel and bladder movements soon set into a pattern that needs no further encouragement.

The trickiest aspect of Its method, most evidently, is training your child without developing a habit of "gifting" every time he/she visits the potty. If your child knows to expect a sweet or small toy at the end of each session, your potty training experience may turn into a series of tantrums and bribes. It is best to avoid handing out ice cream or toy to get your child to sit on the potty. The trick successfully to using Its method is to exercise control over the nature of the rewards you hand out.

Not all rewards for successful urination or bowel movement need to be tangible or edible. Most children, especially during the first three years, are easily delighted and encouraged by nothing more than appreciative laughter, applause, or verbal praise from parents. Many toddlers like their achievements to be noticed; if you're going to turn potty training into an event, ensure that every completion is met with some celebration.

You can keep sweets or other gifts, such as toys or clothing, for more significant potty training milestones. Let your child complete a day of the successful potty session to get a sweet treat after dinner, or take him/her on an underwear shopping trip once the child used the potty successfully for a week or so. You can add to the motivation using such simple tools as stickers and progress charts. For each successful training session, place a sticker on his/her chart – or let the child do it! These little stamps of acknowledgment also serve as the motivation needed to potty train your child.

Three birds with one stone: Teaching potty habits, ownership, and accountability

Toddlerhood is a stage of many discoveries for both you and your child. Your child's first sensations likely recognize those of love, hunger, and happiness – along with the complicated emotion that crankiness brings! Past the first ten to twelve months, the infants then begin grasping such concepts as ownership, responsibility, and accountability for actions. You have to teach them these values at some point – why not tie them into your potty training lessons?

To teach your child ownership, begin by letting him/her choose favorite pairs of underwear. You can either take the child on a shopping trip or have him/her choose from a pile you've already selected. Its simple act should already stir a feeling of responsibility within the child. You notice that he/she may take extra care of these garments; It is a sign that the child has successfully understood ownership and responsibility.

To teach accountability, have him/her wear favorite underwear on the day of your first potty training session. Let the child roam around the house without wearing any diapers, leaving just the underwear to catch any falling feces or urine.

It stages, your child should already have understood the discomfort that It mess can cause. Not wanting to dirty favorite clothes, or feel uncomfortable with a stinky pile of feces or wet urine in his/her pants, your child should be in to sit on the potty.

Its method's success largely depends on your child's response to concepts such as ownership and accountability. If the child has little value for the clothes or does not yet feel uncomfortable with a soiled diaper, it may not be time to introduce Its method to him/her. The right time to teach such concepts, according to many experts, arrives when your child begins asking questions about his/her belongings or starts asserting authority over possessions.

It's a technique to succeed; you also rely on your child's desire to imitate grown-ups' behavior. Children often pick up lessons on ownership from observing their parents' relationship with their belongings. If you make a big show of not dirtying your clothes or visiting the bathroom when it's time, chances are your toddler likely mimic these behavior patterns.

Its method of potty training your child, however, is not without its small share of cons. Teaching anyone – let alone a child – the concept of responsibility is not instantly successful. Your child may take time to connect the mess left by feces and urine and his/her rightful place on the potty as a solution to Its mess. Some other children may, at first, enjoy the mess they create, before becoming aware of its consequences. Still, others may be blissfully oblivious to every lesson you try to impart – be it ownership, cleanliness, or using the potty. More often than not, using its technique may make you feel like you're left with bigger messes to clean up than ever!

What makes its method effective is the amount of patience you exercise throughout the training procedure. At the outset, you have to accept that its robust way of potty training is a messy affair – you have soiled underpants, clothing items, and feces or urine spills to clean from the floor and your child. As exhausting as it may seem initially, and if you want to kill three birds with one stone, persevere with its method. Talk your child through each phase of the potty training, letting him/her understand the importance of its event.

Involve your child in the act of selecting underwear he/she likes. Give your child a compliment in his/her favorite underwear, noting how nice it looks on the child when it's clean. Remind the child, now and again, to let you know when he/she feels like the child is about to urinate. And then, leave the onus of caring for the child's bladder up to him/her! When it's time for the child first to use the potty, you can also exaggerate the process of taking off the underwear, and then cheer loudly once the child has used the potty. Be sure to include praise or two for getting the ownership and accountability concepts right, such as "You used the potty, and your pants are so clean – you're such a good girl/boy!"

Apart from the odd messy incident – or three – you and your child should emerge from It happy and unscathed technique. At most, your child may display signs that he/she is not ready to tackle, taking responsibility for his/her belongings and bowel movements. If it turns out to be the case, you can always try out another method, or take a small break and try again.

Set The Potty Clock – Potty Training Via Routines And Schedules

Since the day of our birth, our bodies help us survive and function by performing specific duties like a well-oiled machine. Such activities as breathing, digesting eaten food, and throwing out waste materials from our bodies need to be undertaken on a timely basis for us to be healthy. To achieve these goals, the body sets its rhythms and patterns of functioning, which best suits the person. Why not take advantage of its daily fixed urination and defecation routine to introduce your child to the potty?

Suppose you don't wish to engage in the messiness that leaving your child in underpants creates, or don't want to make a habit of rewarding your child every time he/she uses the potty. In that case, you may find success in merely guiding your child to the potty when it's time for the daily toilet break. It is a low-fuss method of potty training that does not rely on tricks or tactics, only your child's enthusiasm for routines and achieving goals. Teaching the child that potty breaks are a timely affair that follows a set pattern, you introduce your child to such concepts as structure, schedules, and self-control.

Its method to work, it becomes your responsibility to observe your child's bowel and bladder patterns. Your child should want to defecate during fixed times during the day, with a gap of at least two hours between each potty visit. Its time, your child should also understand the sensations that were wanting to defecate and urinate cause. Once you know the routine, usher him/her toward the potty area and encourage him/her to sit on it at these fixed times.

Sometimes, just the need to release feces or urine at the right time should be enough to get your child going. In other cases, it helps give him/her motivators that are also tied into some form of routine. You could tell of the need to be potty trained in a week or two for a birthday party or family outing, and that these timely potty training sessions are practice. Initially, your child may feel a little pressure, or may only be successful when there is a need to urinate or defecate very urgently. If you are persistent with leading the child to the potty every single time, you can potty train in weeks, even days.

It is a method that works best for those children who show a preference for timetables and display a more goal-oriented nature. If your child likes testing authority and doesn't mind a mess, you may want to consider a more creative technique to potty train. Its routine-based training method is often successful with those children who like being neat and tidy and develop a new understanding of shame and consequence.

It is also a successful method when you, as a parent, can provide plenty of your time, patience, and a consistently stable environment. If you are to potty train your child through routines, you have to introduce him/her to the concept of steady patterns in everyday life. The potty should ideally be in the same spot, so your child knows where to go when it's time. It would help if you led him/her to the potty during every sensation, to familiarize the child with the concept of routine.

Making Good Use Of The Reward System

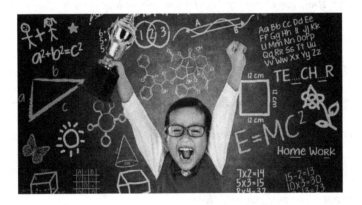

We're talking about a child rather than a puppy, I know, but that doesn't mean the reward system isn't going to be an incredibly effective way of getting its job done. There is nothing quite convincing as a positive reinforcement when it comes to teaching a child the techniques of the world.

Every child is, of course, very different in their temperament and what motivates them. You know your child best, so I leave it to you to decide precisely how you reward them for their success during the potty training phase:

Chapter 9: Simple praise is plenty for many kids. The pride of having done something bright is reinforced with your enthusiastic response, letting him or her know that they have done precisely what they were asked to do, and they've done it right. Let your child know they did it! They did it! They went pee or poop like the big kids! And watch as they burst over with pride and happiness.

Chapter 10: Allow your child to do something that they love doing, but only if they successfully use the potty. Maybe they like it when you let them stir the cookie mixture. Perhaps they want to be the one to turn the bathwater on. In many cases, being allowed to march the potty to the toilet and flush away what they've created is the perfect reward. Little people find great enjoyment in the things we think of as everyday chores – it's all so new to them and exciting. Being given it perceived responsibility as a reward for being all grown up on the potty can be a huge motivator.

Chapter 11: Keep a small reward handy in a box or jar. It could be a sticker or a pin, maybe a fruit roll-up or a healthy snack they like. It should be small but consistent – something you can give your child every time they use the bathroom for the foreseeable future. Some families want to use sticker charts and let their little one fill-up the spaces over time until they have completed it, then give them a big reward they've enjoyed at the end. Some families choose to tell their tot what that prize be; others like it to be a surprise. I tend to err on the side of the first option only because it allows the child to know what they are working towards – and that can be very important, especially if you are working with a little one who is proving more challenging to potty train and need a real boost of motivation to get them there.

Whatever you choose, remember that it is something you be giving or doing for a while – long after the initial success of your potty training weekend. For that reason, it's usually best to avoid rewards such as fried chicken or bars of candy; you are setting yourself up for a long term eating problem!

Then, of course, there is the opposite of a reward: a punishment when your little one doesn't quite get things right. I strongly advocate steering away from anything that would qualify as an actual reprimand.

No early bedtimes, no withholding snacks or toys, nothing like that. It hurt your child's ingress to try, and that is the last thing you want to happen.

In most cases, a simple, "Oh no, you didn't do pee-pee in the potty. That's not where the pee goes, is it?" in a frowny tone of voice is enough to make your point. It lets your child know that he or she has not done what was expected and disapproves of its behavior.

Health And Wellness

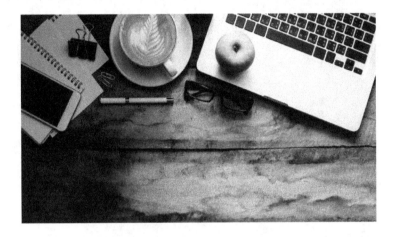

Your goal is to potty train your child, to be sure, but don't lose sight of the rest of the picture. Teaching good hygiene, providing a healthy diet, and offering lots of opportunities to exercise need to be high on your list of priorities. The habits your child develops during potty training may last for years — perhaps for a lifetime.

Hygiene

The habits children develop when learning to use the potty are likely to last a lifetime, so it is essential to teach them to wash their hands and wipe properly and rinse the potty bowl and flush the toilet after each use. It is an excellent time to prepare other etiquette points, such as putting down the toilet seat and lid, wiping up splashes in the sink after hand washing, and straightening the towel before dashing off to play. Toddler boys need to be taught to pay attention when they urinate, so they do not spray the floor and walls and clean up if they do. In general, youngsters need to learn to do their part to help maintain a room where they use lots in the years to come.

Hand Washing

Hand washing does more than keeping toddlers' hands pretty and presentable; it protects them from the disease. Failure to wash hands properly after using the toilet can cause illness — and it often does! Toddlers inevitably get stool on their hands when they wipe themselves, as caregivers when they change diapers and handle soiled laundry. Even traces too small to be seen contain germs. Suppose a contaminated hand has a shortcut or touches the mouth or an eye, bacteria that cause illness to enter the body. Be meticulous about washing your hands after you feel soiled diapers and laundry, and have your child come to you for a clean hands check after he has used the potty by himself.

Wiping

Children do not do an excellent job of cleaning themselves until kindergarten. Besides their lack of practice, their arms are just too short for their bodies. Teach your child to use several small pieces of toilet paper to clean himself, tossing each one as it becomes soiled. It is far more effective than toddlers' natural tendency to use a single big wad. Moistened towelettes can do an even better job, but children need adults to use them at first.

Starting at the vagina, girls should wipe forward with a clean tissue after urinating so as not to get bacteria in the vagina or urethra. For the same reason, they should start just behind the vagina and wipe back along their buttocks after a bowel movement.

Keeping The Penis Clean

You need to make a special effort to keep the penis of an uncircumcised boy clean to reduce the risk of infection. The foreskin of an uncircumcised infant cannot be pulled back, but make it a habit to lift the foreskin gently as soon as it begins to loosen and wash the area carefully during each bath to prevent infection. Please do It by gently wiping with a soft washcloth that has been dipped in warm water, and teach your tot how to do the same when he is old enough. When the foreskin is fully retractable so that it can be folded back over the penis like the cuff of a shirt sleeve over an arm, be sure your child returns it to its normal position after urinating or washing himself. If the foreskin is left folded, it can function as a rubber band. The resulting constriction can cause problems severe enough to require medical treatment.

Diaper Rash

Urine is very acidic and can wreak havoc with delicate baby skin. To help clear up diaper rash, change soiled diapers frequently. Try switching brands of disposables or use cloth diapers. Avoid wipes containing alcohol, drying, and gently blot the skin instead of rubbing it.

Protect against chafing by applying a cream containing zinc oxide. If there is irritation on the sides of the groin or around the waist, fold disposable diapers, so the plastic liners face out and don't touch the skin. It can help a lot to have your child go bare-bottomed for ten minutes to be sure he is dehydrated before putting on a clean diaper. If the rash worsens or persists for three days, it may be a yeast infection, which requires a prescription. See your pediatrician.

Bladder Health

It's not just an old wives' tale that cranberry juice promotes bladder health. Doctors recommend it, too. Drinking lots of water promotes frequent urination, which decreases the risk of bladder infections.

Bladder Infections

Bladder infections are more common in girls because the urethra is short, and in wiping after bowel movements, they can get a bit of stool on the urethral opening. However, boys can and do get bladder infections, too. Bladder infections can increase the frequency of urination and may also create urgency so intense children can't get to the potty in time.

The typical symptom is blood in the urine, which turns it cloudy or pink. There may be a spot of blood on the toilet tissue after urination. Bladder infections can also cause loss of bladder control, frequent and painful urination, the pain just above the pubic area or on the side, fever, and lethargy. They can be severe, so see your doctor fast.

Urinary Tract Infections

Toddler logic has it that what comes out should go in, so most boys use a squeeze bottle or squirt gun in the bathtub and inject some water into the place from which the urine flows. The result can be a urinary tract infection. Be sure to tell your child that he must never put water or anything else in his penis. I hope for the best but be prepared for the worst. Just as toddlers are driven to insert beans in their ears and peas into their nostrils, they are compelled to add water into their penis.

Leakage

Additional leakage after urinating can signal a physical malformation correctable by surgery, so check your child's pants a minute or two after he uses the potty. Otherwise, you might think he had an accident an hour later when he didn't. Also, the stream of urine should be strong and steady. See your doctor if it tends to trickle out or often flows in erratic spurts, even when your child urinates a large quantity. Infants do it, but toddlers should not.

Food Allergies

Food allergies can have adverse bowel and bladder effects, from diarrhea to constipation to bladder irritation. The following are common culprits. Talk to your pediatrician about eliminating them from your child's diet for ten days to two weeks to see if the problem improves, only to recur when the food is eaten once again.

Chapter 12: Milk and dairy products. (Remember that cheese and butter contain milk!)

Chapter 13: Carbonated beverages.

Chapter 14: Artificial colors and sweeteners.

Chapter 15: Citric acid and vitamin C.

Chapter 16: Melons, especially watermelon and cantaloupe.

Chapter 17: Any other foods to which your child is known to be allergic.

Bowel Health

It doesn't matter how often your child has bowel movements. Some only defecate every other day, or even less. Some children have a natural tendency to be constipated. Eating a lot of highly processed (a.k.a. "junk") foods cause constipation because they are absorbed into the system, so ultimately, all that remains is a hard, dense mass. The best cure is a diet rich in fruits, vegetables, and whole grains (especially bran, brown rice, whole wheat, and oats) to add lightweight bulk, and lots of water to soften it. Also, avoid foods that bind, such as bananas, chocolate, peanut butter, and cheese.

Fluid Intake

Toddlers need four to six cups of fluid daily under normal circumstances — more in hot weather or if they are ill with fever, vomiting, or diarrhea. Besides water (from the tap or bottled; plain or carbonated), good sources include soup, juice, and milk. However, milk provides only a cup of fluid per cup; the rest is solids.

Pain and Pressure of Constipation

Severe problems with constipation or worse, with impaction, can complicate potty training. Small hard "marbles" don't usually cause a problem, but full stool can be painful to pass and cause tears that take time to heal. Little drops of blood on underwear or toilet paper may signal that It has happened and rectal itchiness, which occurs as the tears start to heal. Gently wash the anus with soap and water after each bowel movement, and have your youngster soak in a warm bath to ease the pain. Put a dab of petroleum jelly on your finger and insert it into your child's rectum to help protect the sore area.

Psychological Constipation

Emotional factors can undermine children's ability to relax the anal sphincter to release stool, resulting in mental constipation. Sitting on a cold toilet seat, potentially being splashed by cold water (if a potty chair is used), watching part of oneself being discarded and sucked down a noisy drain, and losing the particular time one-on-one time while a beloved parent wipes and cleans and rubs them with sweet-smelling creams and lotions — is it what being a big boy is all about? Stress during potty training can cause constipation. Add to that a diet rich in junk food and low in fiber, and it's no wonder toddlers become constipated.

Diarrhea

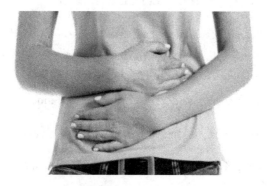

Children don't have much, if any, bowel control during even minor bouts of diarrhea. Put them back in diapers and forget potty training until they're over it. Avoid foods that have a laxative effect, mostly raw fruits, and vegetables, and concentrated fruit juices.

The main risk of diarrhea is dehydration, which is dangerous if it goes on for very long, and can become dangerous very quickly if combined with vomiting and high fever. Taken to an extreme, it is fatal. Lost minerals such as chloride, sodium, and potassium must be replaced quickly. Give your child Gatorade or another electrolyte solution and contact your doctor if you note any signs that serious trouble is brewing: cracked lips, decreased urination, darker or deeper yellow color of urine, urine that appears to have crystals, a sunken soft spot on the head of a young toddler, listlessness, increased pulse.

Penis Health

At birth, the foreskin is fully attached to the penis. It gradually begins to loosen, and by age one, the glans at the tip of the penis itself should be visible. Most boys' foreskin is fully retractable by age four or five, although for a significant percentage, it doesn't occur until much later. At that point, the foreskin can be folded back over the penis to be fully exposed for proper cleaning. The foreskin must never be left folded. That is dangerous and requires an immediate doctor's visit if the penis swells to the point that the foreskin cannot be readily unfolded. Often cold compresses and medications to reduce the swelling are sufficient to return it to normal, but sometimes minor surgery is required to relieve the constriction.

Bedwetting, A Potty-Training Challenge

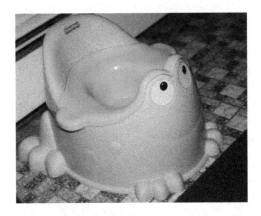

Bedwetting A most likely reason is a developmental delay, biology (even here), sleep disturbance (like sleeping too deep), mental disorders, and psychological, anti-diuretic hormone levels. physiology, Causes of bedwetting

The most often recognized cause of primary nocturnal enuresis, but also the most difficult to prove, is the maturation lag of the central nervous system. Mainly, the infant's nervous system does not believe that the bladder has to be held, and the urine discharges during sleep.

Sleeping conditions affect substantial percentages of children who suffer from bedwetting, and extensive research has been carried out on the matter. Still, the findings have been so varied that it is difficult for researchers to identify a primary sleep disorder that can be defined as the leading cause of litter.

Some people think that bedwetting is primarily behavioral, contributing to the question of emotional concern. Some studies have shown that emotionally, children suffering from nighttime enthusiasts have precisely the same conduct as children who don't. In these studies, that demonstrate psychological distinctions between the two groups, the main differences were that a child with a bedwetting problem was socially less and had most self-esteem problems than the other group. It raises the question: do low self-esteem and social issues go hand in hand with nursing babies or do nursing contribute to these kinds of mental situations?

Family history is essential, and several studies have shown results that it seems almost conclusive that when a parent has had a child's bed weather, their child is likely to have very high chances. One study showed a 77 percent chance in a family in which both parents had the same disease. It helps to dissipate the theory that enuresis is a behavioral problem. It, in effect, makes it more appropriate and induces somewhat less stress and shame, leading to better outcomes following treatment.

Treatment of bedwetting You can try different ways to deal with a bedwetting condition without the intervention of a doctor or medical attention. Whether or not a medical procedure is mainly required depends on many factors: such as the age of a child, how often they wet the bed, and the seriousness perceived by the family of the child. Most children do outgrow bedwetting and need no physician treatment at all for it.

Many parents utilize bedwetting wall pads at night, and although they do a great job in preventing the bed from moisture due to the accident, they do very little to resolve the problem. While concentrating on its aspect of bedwetting is very important, trying to prevent future events is also extremely important. It is why it is good to use many essential methods of prevention as early as possible. So you may decide to take your child to your doctor if they don't function. However, you should know that children under the age of six are generally not treated by doctors if the only problem is bed weeping.

Once you have chosen to bring your child to a doctor about bedwetting, it is essential to know that the ultimate goal of entirely accident-free nights can take a long time to reach. The parent and the child must remain committed to Its long process. There must be two techniques that doctors use to address bedwetting problems: medicine and behavioral therapy. Parents and children must be as cooperative as possible and in to try their doctor's advice. If anyone has a bad attitude, solving the problem can be much more difficult, if not impossible.

The doctor likely wants to remove all medical conditions at the very start. Although most kids seen by doctors are perfectly healthy in bedwetting, some have a medical condition. So, before a doctor approaches it as if they don't, they want to make sure it is true. The doctor's evaluation of your child should be targeted to exclude anatomical abnormalities of urinary bladder or tract. These may involve conditions like postural urethral valves, an ectopic ureter, or an episodic urethra that is an opening of the urethra of the penis' dorsum. When the doctor undertakes a thorough examination, which involves a family medical history, physical examination, and urine analysis, he or she can usually determine whether there is a medical condition and, if so, what the disorder could be. If your child is treated for enuresis and even before, it is an excellent idea to keep a record of incidents of bedwetting. In addition to its dairy, it is great to write down anything that could have occurred that day to disturb the child's natural emotional equilibrium if the bedwetting of the baby does not happen repetitively at night.

When you determine whether or not there is a medical condition that contributes to your child's bedwetting situation, you can see which methods of treatment help you best. It is worth noting that coherent take-up could be a key to improving bed weathering (it is also worth knowing that most doctors usually describe improvements as a decline in bedwetting regularity of 50%).

Your physician may choose to use only one or both methods of treatment together. The therapeutic strategies may and typically include an alarm system, a recompense system, demand for your child to switch sheets, and bladder training.

Bedwetting alarms can be a useful tool to help your baby retrain the sleep patterns so that he or she sleep better and wake up a little more often during the night. You can schedule them for some time to get your child up and try to use it anytime the alarm goes off.

A reward system can also be a useful behavioral therapy tool, particularly when the child has developed new patterns of sleep and has less frequent injuries. Giving a small bonus each day after a dry night or a large prize at the end of a particular duration, including a whole week of dry nights, can give your child even more incentive to wake up at night.

Changing the bedding for your baby is also a great way to prevent them from getting as many bedding nights. Although it's not fair to punish a child for anything they can't control, it is not punishment, and it's a way for them to understand that, even when they are asleep, they have to take responsibility for their actions. It also works well because they have to get out of bed and sleep more often, which can, in effect, make them sleep better regularly.

One type of behavioral therapy is bladder training, which can help reduce bed weeping nights. That is because your child holds its bladder for longer and longer periods during the day. You may always go to the toilet when you feel the urge to go, and so when you fall into a deep sleep, your body reacts when it reaches you. When you teach your child to keep it for as long as they can when the urge arrives while awake, they are more likely to be able to resist it subconsciously while asleep.

If behavioral therapy does not work and medicines can only be prescribed if the child is seven years old. Medications work best in behavioral treatment, as it is not a bedwetting solution. They can also have side effects. If you decide to use drugs to treat your child, there are two common types, one prescribed by your doctor. One helps the bladder to maintain more urine and reduces the urine in the kidneys. These are not the kinds of medication you want your child to use regularly across their lives.

It's not only you'll try to help your child overcome their bedwetting dilemma, but you should also focus on assisting them in understanding it and, if possible, don't feel so bad about it. Your child probably feels very ashamed of being in bed. You may also feel guilty that you can't control your body in the way you think you can. For older children, it is very likely. It's a problem; you should never punish your child. It is essential to remember that your baby can not prevent it. The older the child is, the more so, and your child is probably more irritated than you are. You try not to make your child feel guiltier of it than they do.

It can also help your child know that nobody knows the cause of bedwetting exactly because each case has too many factors to consider. Tell them about the many various objects that could impact their condition and the fact that they are not responsible for these reasons, and that you help them overcome it. Tell them all the knowledge they need to help them do so without thinking less of themselves. For example, when you wet the bed as a baby, be sure to explain and remind them that it could run in families. It could help to relieve some of the pressure and some of your remorse.

Remember, it's hard for you and your child to use any means necessary to clean up your bedwetting problems. The correct no-fault attitude can help and open your mind to treatment suggestions and be committed to any way you decide to treat sleeping weathering and potty training

Cross-Cultural And Historical Approaches To Potty Training

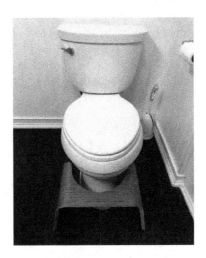

Having an understanding of how toilet training takes place in other parts of the world can help inform and reassess one's ideas about its topic. Accounts of successful infant toileting approach worldwide attest to the first bladder and bowel capabilities of babies and show that in most places, toddler toilet training is not the norm. Perhaps you be surprised or inspired by what you read.

In the majority of those places, there is often a preference for traditional toileting methods; but the high cost or limited availability of disposable diapers can also be a factor. Thus, potty training methods that have been practiced for generations are still alive and in widespread use. In other parts of the world, such as the former Soviet Union, where the use of disposable diapers has become commonplace, only portions of the population have retained more traditional toileting methods.

Though potty training practices around the world have not been fully or widely documented, a few scientific studies offer detailed and reliable descriptions of approaches used in specific cultures. In places where lessons have not been conducted, we can turn to descriptive articles and anecdotal evidence to gain an understanding of traditional training methods used.

East Africa

Digo mothers have high expectations for their babies' capabilities and infant behavior. They begin elimination communication in the first weeks after birth and expect that by 3 to 5 months in age, their babies possess a "high degree of motor and social development." They also hope that by 4 to 6 months, babies be reasonably dry both in the daytime and at night. Using graduated expectations, babies are trained to not only manage their toileting by age one but also to be independent and self-sufficient enough to be left in the care of other community members while the mother is working.

During the first two months of life, Digo babies spend all of their time in close physical contact with their mothers, who take responsibility for all training. Traditionally, babies are worn in slings, allowing mothers to go about their daily tasks with free hands. Digo mothers believe that understanding and responding to all their babies' needs is a crucial part of infant development as it fosters a baby's sense of security. Through constant physical contact, Digo mothers develop an understanding of when their infants need to eliminate.

In its approach, mothers use both physical and sound associations to foster bladder and bowel control, differentiating for urination or passing stool. When a baby needs to urinate, his mother sits on the ground with her legs straight and lays the baby on her shins facing up, holding him by his bent knees. She also makes a "shuus" sound. After the infant has peed, there is a reward in the form of a feed, a cuddle, or another close contact. For bowel movements, the mother sits and bends her knees to make a "seat" on her feet for the child, who is placed facing her. She does not make a sound association for bowel movements. When the baby wakes up from a nap, has just eaten, or only when the mother senses it is time for elimination, the mother takes her infant to an outside training spot.

Digo Bladder Training Posture

Toilet training that "can't be done" (90-day old infant)

Photo and caption: Prof. Dr. Marten W. deVries, Digo Society, Kenya. 1974

Digo Bowel Training Posture

Photo: Prof. Dr. Marten W. deVries, Digo Society, Kenya. 1974

Between 3 and 5 months of age, other community members begin to take part in toileting the babies. Interestingly, it is usually 5-to 12-year-old girls who take on the role of helpers. According to the authors, day or night-time accidents during the first year are treated casually. However, after the age of 1, there is an expectation that a Digo toddler takes himself independently to a designated spot outside the house to urinate and have a bowel movement. Accidents and regression among toddlers were uncommon.

The anthropologists note that the Digo people consider their babies to be active rather than passive participants in toilet training.

Digo people's lifestyles, living conditions, clothing, and family roles are all very different from that of modern societies. At the same time, it field study demonstrates that it is entirely physically possible for a 1-year-old to be potty trained. I found it fascinating to read that mothers maintained such a firm conviction about the potential and capabilities of infants. The Digo people believe that the first year of life is a vital time for teaching and shaping an infant's ways, mainly through constant feedback, being in tune with their child, and regularly communicating with and responding to the child throughout the day. A 1999 study by MW deVries looked at the precocity of African babies and noted a positive correlation to traditional environments and a mother's diet during pregnancy and breastfeeding. The Digo babies, who were kept in close physical contact with a career while awake and asleep, frequently stimulated and fed on demand, achieved developmental milestones earlier than their European or American counterparts. In many ways, it "ancient" thinking is becoming new, modern thought. In recent years, 'attachment parenting' and baby-wearing have become more common and even fashionable.

Vietnam

A recent series of papers by Duong and colleagues examined potty training practices in Vietnam and also compared findings with a cohort of potty training Swedish children. One of the documents entitled "Vietnamese mothers' experiences with potty training procedure for children from birth to 2 years of age" described and documented traditional practices in Vietnam. All 47 children in the study were potty trained by age 2, with most being able to use their potties by nine months. By age 2, the children could independently manage all their toileting needs (Duong, 2012).

The traditional method used was a variation of Elimination Communication. A critical factor in developing bowel and bladder control was a whistling sound made by the mothers, which signaled the baby to void. The mothers also checked the children frequently for indications or signs that they needed to eliminate.

Ongoing communication between the mother and baby played a significant part in potty training success.

Thailand

A 2011 study from Thailand resonated most with my potty training endeavors. Though the authors' objective was to examine the age at which Thai babies begin and complete toilet training and associated factors (Benjasuwantep, 2011), the description of the Thai toileting method was also quite significant.

The method used was dubbed "assisted toilet training." The study's authors write that though Elimination Communication techniques used in Thailand are similar to those practiced by the Digo people (with perhaps less rigidity as to age-appropriate expectations), the age of starting potty training was somewhat later with its particular cohort. Of the 50 infants who participated, about 92% began toilet training between four months and one year. 60% began training after the age of 6 months. Almost half of all the babies observed were successfully prepared by one year of age. Some caregivers used a potty while others started by holding their child over a potty or other designated spot.

The majority of parents in the study (74%) potty trained by watching for signs that their child was about to eliminate, and a smaller portion of parents (26%) used a schedule with set times to place their children on the potty.

China

Many visitors to China are struck by the sight of toddlers running around in open-crotch or split pants, known locally as kaidangku, which allow them to squat and eliminate at their convenience.

China is another country where Elimination Communication is still widely practiced, though disposable diaper usage has steadily increased over the past few decades, particularly at nighttime. Traditionally, babies are toileted in the first few months of life by parents or grandmothers using methods similar to those we read about above. There have been many reports of babies adopted from China arriving at their new homes in the West already potty trained; it means that caregivers in orphanages had been potty training groups of children simultaneously.

According to Chinese practice, once a baby can stand, he is taught to squat to eliminate. Though potties are used at home and daycares, Chinese children squat to eliminate when out of the house. Its practice can be witnessed in playgrounds or other public spaces, including on public transportation.

After the age of 12-14 months, children are generally expected to manage their own toileting needs, though they may be assisted with It. In many larger cities, its practice is becoming less widespread due to efforts to keep cities cleaner, to family income increases, and according to some, to successful ad campaigns by diaper companies.

Ukraine

In Ukraine and other post-Soviet countries, disposable diapers were not widely available until after the fall of the Soviet Union in 1991. While commonly used now, their relatively high cost means that many modern parents continue to potty-train their children early to save money by avoiding diaper costs. According to one recent article, 40% of mothers begin training when their babies are 6-8 months old (Ukrsbaby, 2017).

While there is no commonly known traditional Ukrainian infant potty training approach, a casual observer notice babies and toddlers at playgrounds being taken aside to tree-lined areas at regular intervals to pee. In the case of babies, you may hear parents making a sound such as "pss, pss" to establish a sound association. While some parents (I have seen it done by mothers and fathers alike) seem to use its technique instinctively, others are oblivious to it. Some parents begin potty training at six months, while others start closer to 2. In any case, most Ukrainian children are out of diapers between 18 months and 2 ½ years of age.

USA & Europe - Historical Approaches

American parents have followed different trends in potty training from the beginning of the 20th century. At one point, the advice included enforcing strict elimination schedules and using aggressive toilet training methods, while at other times, gentle early training more reminiscent of Elimination Communication was typical. Many believe that it was the forceful and strict potty training that prompted the switch to a laxer attitude; it coincided with the invention of disposable diapers.

Making The Results Stable

We'll take you through how you can maintain your progress and methods to use under various circumstances.

In A Car

Potty training in a car can be quite challenging as the child is away from the familiar environment. Whether you are on a short journey or a long road trip, it is essential to prepare for the inevitable as the child may need to ease yourself. Though Its situation might be different for you and the child, adaptability is critical.

Some parents choose to use diapers when on a road trip. We don't need advice; you do it, as it is moving back to square one. However, you can use diapers if your child is still very new to potty training.

There are other ways you can prepare yourself and the child for road trips. First, you should prepare yourself mentally for any possibility. Do not get surprised if the child suddenly says he has to pee. Before leaving the house, let the child know you are going on a ride and encourage him to empty his bowels if he needs to. Communication is an essential aspect of potty training. It is necessary to carry the child along in whatever decision you are about to make.

To continue with potty training, even when in a car, there are some necessary supplies you need to aid the process if you do not want to use diapers. The first thing you should get is a travel potty, which always is in the car, along with wipes and disinfectants. You can also use the travel potty in public toilets if you do not want your child to sit in a public bathroom. If you have no other choice, get disposable toilet seat covers for extra protection.

Getting disposable bags is also recommended. You can store the child's clothes in them in case of accidents and also use it to dispose of the child's waste. It also prevents any mess from dropping into the car. Ensure the child is dressed in easily removable clothes in case of an urgent need to go.

Have a clean towel always ready in case of accidents. To reduce the frequency of accidents, make sure you stop at intervals at places such as gas stations or stores to give the child a chance to ease himself. You can also bring extra clothes, car seat covers, and extra underwear along to be safe.

In A Daycare

Maintaining the potty training results when a child goes to daycare requires the cooperation of the parent and the daycare provider. The real challenge is the change in environment and bathroom routine.

In the past, most daycares used to offer to help potty train children, but such daycares are hard to find these days, if not non-existent. Nowadays, most daycares only accept potty-trained children or prefer to let the child use diapers instead of going commando.

You should take a tour of the daycare first to make sure the environment is clean and safe enough for the child. Thoroughly inspect the facilities and ask questions when necessary.

It is essential to take time to read the daycare policy and discuss it with the provider before registering your child to prevent issues. After getting a daycare with a suitable potty training policy, you can check the terms and then sign the agreement.

To make it convenient for both the child and the daycare provider, discuss the potty training method the child uses at home and the bathroom routine with the provider. You can also consider the reward system and the usual toilet facilities the child is used to. Also, inform the caregiver that be in charge of your child about the typical signs that the child is about to go. It is essential, as the child may be reluctant to speak to an unfamiliar face.

We advise you to make sure the child is comfortable with the caregiver. Let the child know he can talk to the caregiver if he needs to go.

If your child can only use a potty chair at the moment, you can bring the child's potty along if the provider is comfortable with it. Using the same equipment makes it easier for the child to adjust. Bring extra clothes and underwear for the child in case of accidents.

You can request reports and feedback from the provider periodically to know about the child's progress.

In A Public Place

To maintain potty training results when with your child in a public place, we advise you to create a potty plan before leaving your home. Preparation is vital to sustaining the progress you've made. You must be mentally prepared as your child may need to use the toilet at any time.

Before leaving the house, let your child ease himself if he needs to. You can try it many times before leaving. If the destination is a familiar place, make a mental note of where the nearest bathroom is or places where you can quickly stop along the way, such as gas stations, stores, or restaurants.

When in public, don't get too carried away to pay attention to your child when he needs to use it. You can develop a safe word or physical signal with your child, which can be used in public to know when the child needs to use it.

Don't panic if the child shows signs that he is about to go or says so. Calmly move the child to the nearest bathroom and try to distract him on the way there. Always choose bathrooms that are mostly unoccupied or less noisy.

Making The Results Stable For Boys

It is commonly said that boys take a little while to get potty trained. It is not a proven fact, but regardless, there are ways you can ensure you keep getting results.

If the child has older male siblings, you can let him watch and imitate them. For example, tell him he gets to wear the same type of "grown-up" underwear as Daddy if he cooperates. If the child still pees in a potty and thinks it's time to move to the toilet, let him watch how his brothers use the bathroom and, since kids learn primarily by imitation, he'll want to try that too.

You can let the child pee while sitting down, and when he becomes comfortable, you can motivate him to go like Daddy. You can add stickers in the toilet for him to aim at.

With every accomplishment, praise the child for motivating him to do more, e.g., "You're a big boy now," or "Tell Dad what you did today." Shop for attractive underwear with him and encourage him not to soil his 'big boy' underwear.

For Girls

Some experts believe it is easier to maintain potty training results for girls, as they begin a little earlier and are easy to train than boys. However, making the results stable requires consistency and overall patience.

Always try your best to maintain the usual bathroom routines and habits. If any change must be introduced, do it gradually, as a sudden change can confuse your child.

Let your child have her favorite doll with her when using her potty. You can also let the child observe her big sister or Mommy use the toilet. It is advisable to use cotton underwear instead of switching to diapers, though you'll have more clean-up.

The most important thing is to maintain a positive environment. If accidents happen, do not overreact, but instead try to find the cause and look for ways to get back on track. Make sure to repeat the potty training instructions and routine to the child and let her recite them.

Another way of ensuring the results are stable is to let the child acquire some independence in using the bathroom. Teach the child how to wipe herself correctly (from front to back) and wash her hands after she's done. With time, these processes become a habit, and accidents are very infrequent.

Potty Training Siblings: Learning Together And Separately

If you have more than one child undergoing potty training at the same time, you might need some extra work and motivation to make sure you maintain results. To an extent, the children should be able to learn together, but you should note that even though they are siblings, the same method may not work for both of them. You'll have to be consistent in whichever ways you adopt. However, you can use its situation to your advantage, depending on how you approach it, as the children can positively influence each other. Depending on the circumstance, you can either let them learn together or separately.

The first thing is to get separate potty chairs for the children. You won't want a kind of situation where both children need to go at the same time with only one potty available. If you want the kids to learn separately, doing it is also necessary. Let each kid have their potty chair, which should be easily identifiable. The same goes for underwear and training pants.

Suppose the children are at different stages of potty training. In that case, you should train them separately for a while, as two things have the possibility of happening: the kids either learn from each other, or one of them might be affected negatively, which may lead to regression. However, if the siblings are at the same stage of potty training, it can work to your advantage as they can learn from each other. They'll be motivated by each other's progress, making the process easier for all the parties involved.

For Kids After Four Years Old

Maintaining potty training results for kids after the age of four should be more comfortable, especially if the child started potty training at an early age. However, the child can still experience accidents at any age, though they vary in frequency.

As a parent, you should learn to pay attention to your child's physical and emotional well-being. Sudden changes can cause the child to get disturbed emotionally, which could lead to anxiety and cause potty training accidents. The child may wet himself either as a result of stress or neglect by the parent. Shaming the child when potty accidents occur can also affect the child's confidence and result in more mistakes.

In all, communication is vital in maintaining the potty training results. Let the child feel free to express his feelings and try to help solve any issues.

Toilet Training A Child With Special Needs

Potty training is one of the toddlerhood's most significant developmental milestones. When your child can graduate from diapers to underwear, a new sense of independence and accomplishment emerge. Children with disabilities (developmental, learning, physical, and behavioral) may need some adjustments to their daily schedules and the overall potty-training plan to achieve their goal. Never assume that a child with learning disabilities or special needs remain incontinent.

Potty-Training Readiness

It is essential to take another look at the steps necessary for successful potty training to have a clear map to guide you when determining your child's readiness. The first step your child must demonstrate is the ability to feel the urge to urinate and have bowel movements. Its capacity is typically first seen in children between the ages of fifteen and twenty-four months. In children with special needs, however, these signs may come somewhat later.

The next step involves your child mastering the ability to hold in urine or stool. Your child being able to stay dry for at least two hours may demonstrate its skill. The ability to keep dry or "hold it" is usually seen around twenty-six to twenty-nine months but maybe later for children of special needs. You may observe your child doing the potty dance, squatting down on her heels, or standing very still with her buttocks squeezed together. It can be frustrating for parents who mistake these cues as attempts to avoid going to the potty. On the contrary, when these behaviors are observed, parents should be encouraged that their little one can hold urine or stool.

The next step is to ensure that your child can get to the potty with minimal assistance. She must then be able to pull down her pants and underwear and sit on the potty (seat or chair). The ability to sit on the toilet usually occurs around twenty-six to thirty-one months of age. In children of special needs, it may occur at a later age. Once on the toilet or potty chair, your child must relax and either urinate or defecate. She is not able to have a bowel movement if she is unable to relax. Please focus on the posture your child assumes on the potty because It is related to her ability to relax. Remember, a step stool may be necessary for children who are too short of reaching the floor with their feet.

Potty Training The Child With ADHD

Attention-Deficit/Hyperactivity Disorder (ADHD) is a neurological disease found in 4 to 7 percent of children and affects boys more often than girls. Children are not typically diagnosed with their condition until after they have reached school age. To arrive at its diagnosis, children must meet several criteria. Symptoms must be present in more than one setting (e.g., home and school), observed before age seven. They must contribute to deficits in schoolwork, the accomplishment of tasks, and overall impairment of performance. Other disorders or conditions frequently coexist with ADHD, including depression, anxiety disorder, oppositional defiant disorder, and tics. Although ADHD is not usually made until the school-age years, some children may show symptoms while still preschool age. ADHD presents differently for each child; some children may show only mild inattention while others are incredibly inattentive and have the hyperactive component as well.

Helping Your Child With ADHD

A refusal to use the toilet or your child's inability to carry out the steps you've been working on may be partially attributed to oppositional defiance or anxiety and an attention deficit. Although you may become very frustrated with your child when she refuses to use the potty, your emotions must remain neutral. Children with oppositional defiance or anxiety disorders only worsen if parents show outward signs of anger, frustration, and stress. Treat accidents lightly. Also, remember to go at your child's pace when potty training. Be sure to give encouragement and praise for each success. You can also prevent or reduce your child's anxiety by beginning potty training at low-stress levels. Avoid times of change, such as with the birth of a new baby, a divorce, or a move to a new home. If you find yourself already in the middle of training and realize the impact a life change or stressor has had on your child, it is always okay to abandon efforts for now and resume once family routines become normalized.

Potty Training Children With Autism Spectrum Disorders

Asperger's syndrome and autism spectrum disorders belong to a group of ailments known as Pervasive Developmental Disorders (PD.D.). Autism spectrum disorders affect between 1 in 80 and 1 in 240 children in the United States, according to the Centers for Disease Control. The conditions across all racial, ethnic, and socioeconomic groups and affect boys almost five times more often than girls.

Challenges For Training

Recent surveys of parents of children with autism show more than 50 percent reporting problems with potty training. Further reports indicate that approximately 11 percent have urinary accidents, while almost 7 percent have stooling accidents. The issues faced by children with autism are more often related to the struggles caused by them being unable to perform developmentally appropriate tasks at their chronological age. Due to language delays and challenges with communication, children with autism may have difficulty understanding instructions and verbalizing the need to go to the potty.

Helping Your Child With Autism Spectrum Disorders

One way to minimize the challenges of potty training a child with autism spectrum disorders is by choosing a method that suits your child's developmental abilities. Its point, you have likely invested a good deal of time in establishing your child's readiness. For example, you have spent time with your child choosing a potty seat or chair that he is likely to use. A child with autism may require additional help as you begin to go through the steps of potty training due to his struggles with communication. One system that you may find beneficial for giving visual cues to your child is the Picture Exchange Communication System. Its structure includes several drawings that are used to educate children with autism. Once you begin the toilet training process, you want to have his teachers or caregivers in the plan since they can provide the toileting prompts and reinforcements during the day. It is important to remember that you are not alone in the process of toilet training your child with an autism spectrum disorder.

Potty Training Children With Sensory Integration Dysfunction

Sensory integration dysfunction, also known as sensory processing disorder, is a diagnosis that refers to a glitch in the system of taking in stimulus, processing it, and responding to it. Sensory integration begins before birth and continues throughout life. However, the most crucial development occurs before a child reaches the age of seven. When a neural processing system is working according to plan, the neurological system (sight, sound, taste, touch, and smell) receives a message, the brain sorts, and filters it. The body or person uses the information to adapt to the environment. Adapting to the environment is how children develop "normally."

Helping Your Child With Sensory Integration Disorder

You need to recognize the symptoms of sensory processing disorder to create an environment that minimizes the frustration or anxiety related to potty training. As a parent, you must first understand that your potty-training experiences with its child be markedly different than those experiences with unaffected children and those of your peers. It is crucial to wait until your child's developmental age is appropriate for potty training. Remember, her chronological age is not relevant here. Experts recommend using a child-oriented approach when potty training a child with a sensory processing disorder.

Potty Training Children With Physical Disabilities

Children with physical disabilities are frequently slower to potty train than children without physical limitations. Sometimes It may be due to accompanying learning disabilities that prevent them from understanding or remembering the steps to going to the potty. They may have difficulty sensing bowel and bladder fullness or the urge to potty. Also, they may have trouble with the physical act of getting to the potty, pulling down their pants, sitting on the potty, and wiping. And lastly, they may have difficulty communicating the need to potty.

Helping Your Child With Physical Disabilities

It is essential to assess the physical aspect of how your child sits on the potty. If upper body strength or posture is a problem, a parent may need to sit with the child to stabilize him while he uses the potty. However, if upper body strength is not an issue, and modifications such as grab bars have already been installed, parental presence is unnecessary. It further promotes your child's progress toward independence.

Raised toilet seats and safety bars are an excellent option for children who are older and taller. For toddlers, however, several potty chairs are commercially available with backs that support posture.

Potty Training Children With Mental Retardation And Down Syndrome

Children who have an intelligence quotient (IQ) less than 70 and have an impaired ability to function are considered to have mental retardation. Children with Down syndrome often fall into It category as well. A diagnosis of mental retardation or global developmental delay is given to preschool-age children when they consistently fail to meet developmental milestones at the projected chronological ages. The signs are usually encountered in order but at a rate slower than their peers. Children with an IQ of 70 may expect to potty train around age three, while children with an IQ of 50 may be closer to the age of four before potty training.

Smearing

Children with mental retardation and autism spectrum disorders may display a behavior known as smearing. Smearing is just as you may imagine—the child smears stool on herself, creating a feeling of satisfaction (for the child, of course). Some children engage in its behavior as an attention-seeking act, while others smear to express their agitation. Some children merely do it out of boredom. Children who spread stool are often unaware of how inappropriate the activity is in the social setting.

Helping Your Child With Mental Retardation

Assisting the child with Down syndrome and mental retardation is centered on improving communication. If verbal communication is a problem for your child, it is essential to devise an alternate way to communicate. Hand signals or pointing to a picture are potential solutions. Remember, each caregiver, teacher, and daycare worker must know the message or have the same image to be consistent in the training process. It is paramount that you remain patient as you embark on the potty-training journey. Keep a positive attitude.

The Three Days Of Training To Go To Potty Training.

After completing preparations for the three-day workout, the weekend begins!

<u>Day 1</u>

The most crucial thing you do today is wake up as soon as you know your son is awake. Assuming your child stays and plays quietly in his room and usually goes back to sleep, it is no longer an option. We want to start the day with the actions we want your child to start taking.

We want to start teaching the habit of using the bathroom as soon as the child wakes up. The only way it can happen is to get up as soon as you hear your child.

If you sleep soundly and know the average time your baby usually wakes up, you should set the alarm before that. You must be awake and ready from the moment your child wakes up. If your body and that of your baby can handle it, it should be a day of salty foods that pushes many fluids. In a nutshell, we need to create the urge to urinate as often as possible.

You and your partner must do the same. You can use your child's favorite drink or press for drinking lots of water.

Be careful not to let your baby drink so much that his stomach hurts. The goal is to do it with the least frustration and stress possible. You should take your baby to the bathroom every 15-30 minutes to try to urinate or defecate during the day. That's why it's essential to cancel the program.

If you have a smartphone, you can use the timer to remind you or download a free training application to remember when it's time to go to the bathroom. Whenever you or your partner has to go to the toilet, the child should go to the bathroom. It allows them to continue learning the steps to use the bathroom. It also helps if you record the steps involved.

First step

Chapter 18: *"Oh! I have to pee or poop. It's time to go to the bathroom."*

Second step

Chapter 19: *Lower your pants.*

Third step

Chapter 20: *Take your panties off later.*

Fourth phase

Chapter 21: *Now, sit in the bathroom to use it.*

Phase five

Chapter 22: *Do you hear that sound? Is pee or poop what comes out of my body?*

Step six

Chapter 23: It is time to clean.

Step seven

Chapter 24: Time to lift my panties.

Step eight

Chapter 25: Upload my pants.

Step nine

Chapter 26: It's time to empty the potty.

Step ten

Chapter 27: Now is the time to wash my hands with warm soapy water.

It is essential to use the right words to explain what your body does. They must know and understand that these things are every day.

Whenever your child pees or poo successfully in the bathroom, even if he's very young, it's time to celebrate. Please put on your special trivial dance and reward your child with a sticker or prize they decide to use. Remember that the goal is not necessarily for a child to learn to associate a reward with using the bathroom.

Verbal praise can be as easy as saying what a great job they did when used the bathroom. You can strengthen it by telling them how smart and "big" they are because they used the potty.

Statistics have shown that about ten times more effective in using the bathroom, children begin to associate what they are doing (pee or poop) with the bathroom.

It is essential to stick to it even in the event of an accident. Children, floors, furniture, and clothes can be washed.

If an accident occurs, that's fine. Clean it and continue. If your child has an accident, you should keep in mind that what you have done is correct.

Of course, it should give a sense of tranquility that, although they made a mistake, is still loved and accepted. Remind them gently but firmly that you need to urinate and defecate in the bathroom.

It is important not to yell at your child or try to be ashamed of him when accidents occur. It is an excellent modification for your baby. The child can and should help clean up any accidents.

They don't, and they shouldn't do it alone. Put a hand on your head while cleaning the mess.

It is perfectly acceptable to wear a diaper or to get up during a nap and before bedtime. Take them to the bathroom before going to bed or sleeping. It creates the habit of using the bathroom before bedtime. Over time, it reduces the amount of moisture during sleep. Once the baby wakes up regularly, you can start letting him sleep without a diaper.

<u>Day 2</u>

Today we add something new to the routine that we follow the first day. We also give you some fun a day. We are sure that you and your child are probably tired of being at home every day.

After completing your morning routine, start facing the day, as usual, respecting yesterday's schedule.

At some point in the day, immediately after using the potty, announce that since they used the potty, it is time to go out and play. When the weather is terrible, think of a fun indoor activity. Today you can go out to play or have fun with indoor activities as a reward for using the bathroom. You saw your baby. Wear underwear and not a diaper.

Stay close to home and bring extra clothes in case of an accident. Play outside or participate in an indoor activity for an hour.

The actual goal is to teach your child to use the bathroom when asked to use the bathroom. It's like when we were children, and our parents told us to use the bathroom before traveling by car. If, during your game, your child indicates that he must use the bathroom, stop the activity immediately, and take him to the bathroom. If you play outdoors in your backyard and have a privacy fence, you can make one of your training holes.

Indeed, you should only do it if the weather is warm enough, and there is enough privacy for your child. But, your child may not tell you if you should use the bathroom. Pay attention to the signs the bathroom should use. Some signs your child can show to indicate that they should use the potty:

Watch for massive changes in your child's facial expressions. It is especially true if the child needs to defecate. You can look for signs of tension.

Your baby can grab the genitals if he needs to urinate—every time your child takes his genitals.

Say, "Let's use the bathroom." Please stop what you are doing at the moment and take them to use the potty. They may be angry because the activity must be enjoyable. Assure them that they are well and that they can continue their business after using the bathroom. Therefore, be sure to follow.

Remember to keep things stress free. Do not use harmful words or guilt on the second day.

In case of an accident, follow the advice provided for the first day. Work with your child to clean it and remind him that pee and poop belong only to the potty.

<u>Day 3</u>

It is his third and last day of intense training to go to the bathroom. You and your child have worked very hard over the past two days. Today it is no different, but now he continues to acquire the habit of using the bathroom.

You want to continue your routine from day 1. Today is different because you go out more than once. Plan your time outdoors according to the weather and your daily activities.

Before leaving each time, tell your child the plan and take him to use the potty first. Remember, you can use the license as a reward for using the bathroom.

The two times you go out, you want to dress them completely. Part of learning to use the potty is to lower pants and underwear and lift them. The only way to understand that action is to do it firsthand. It also builds independence. If you have a baby bath, use it on the second and third days. If you have a private patio, you can use one of the training holes inside your home.

Today is simply a day when you become stronger and continue using the potty at regular intervals. Tell your child to use the bathroom. It's okay to wear them and help them with their clothes and make them feel too.

While venturing twice today, it continues to reinforce that we have to maintain our urge to urinate or defecate until we can get to the bathroom.

Again, it is something that can take some time to learn. Some children cannot keep up with others. That is why it is crucial not to go too far from your home or go to the bathroom. You want to foster a feeling of skill and independence.

After training, make sure they have a bare bottom for at least three months inside the house. Note that if trained babies wear diapers again, they become too relaxed and lazy.

They believe diapers are a type of substitute and begin to urinate and defecate, which frustrates the purpose of the workout. When you go out, make them wear loose pants without underwear and diapers.

Bring a portable chair with you if you need to take it for a long trip. If your child has not been successful in training, do not demoralize him. He failed several reasons, such as incorrect training age, stressful environment, improper monitoring, et al.

Sometimes, all the factors are perfect, and even in their case, the child may fail, also if it does not happen frequently.

Don't talk about training in front of the baby for at least 6-8 weeks. Its time, you can restart the workout.

CONCLUSION

Thank you for reading all this book!

You should always come back and read this book, especially if you feel lost or need more guidance to help you through difficult or decisive moments. I'm sure that if you have finished reading this book and you are on your way to starting the potty training, chances are you will find this whole process easier. I have given you tools that are effective, straightforward, and, above all, functional.

"Okay, so; I have read this book now; where can I start?" because sometimes it may feel like there's too much information given at once. I was in that precise position as well, and I felt like nobody understood me!

However, I would like to encourage you to listen to your motherly or fatherly instincts, and to know that you should start by recognizing that potty training is a process. It will take time, dedication, love, commitment, and trust if you want to accomplish your goal to have a fully potty trained toddler.

Lastly, it doesn't matter if you have tried potty training before, and you have failed; because the truth is, the only thing that matters now is that you have allowed yourself to discover this guide, and you can easily replicate these steps on your own.

Rest assured that someone else has done it this way before you, and it was a complete success!

I wish you a loving, peaceful, and not-too-messy potty training journey! And hopefully, this will be the end of the diapers in your household!

You have already taken a step towards your improvement.

Best wishes!